Intermittent Fasting and Autophagy

A Step by Step Beginners Guide for Weight Loss, Build Muscle, Detox Your Body and Boost Your Energy Through the Process of Metabolic Autophagy (for Women and Men)

Dorothy Smith

Table of Contents

Introduction

Thank you so much for purchasing the book *Intermittent Fasting and Autophagy: A Step by Step Beginners Guide for Weight Loss, Build Muscle, Detox Your Body and Boost Your Energy Through the Process of Metabolic Autophagy for Women and Men*. In this book, we will give you a piece of guided information on how you can not only lose fat but gain muscle at the same time.

As you might know, intermittent fasting has to be one of the best ways to achieve optimal success in regards to health and wellness, which is why understanding how you should follow this diet plan is fundamental. To give you a little breakdown, we will be going through how to autophagy, and intermittent fasting goes hand in hand. We will also cover the benefits which come along following autophagy.

Finally, we will also help you understand why it is so important to eat certain foods to see an enhanced benefit from fasting. We will talk briefly about the ketogenic diet and the alkaline diet. And how it can help you to see better results from following these eating plans. With that being said, we have made this book very easy to follow along. We have also made things very congruent, meaning you will have no trouble understanding the concept behind each eating plan and how the results you have been looking for can be achieved. One thing to remember will be to follow everything in this book if your goal is to maximize your results.

Chapter 1: Intermittent Fasting and Autophagy

Welcome to the first chapter, in this chapter, we will talk about intermittent fasting and autophagy and how do they compare with each other. The truth is that to achieve autophagy, you need to go through intermittent fasting. Intermittent fasting, as you know, is one of the best ways to not only detoxify your body but to lose fat and build muscle. Building upon that, intermittent fasting is also shown to detoxify your body in a tremendous amount. This is why intermittent fasting can not only provide you with health benefits but also give you amazing results aesthetically. If you do not know what intermittent fasting is, then we will go through that in a little bit. But first, let me give you a brief on how intermittent fasting started. Intermittent fasting started to change up things; it was first known as The Warrior Diet. This is where people would not eat for 20 hours, and would only have four hours to eat. Even though many bodybuilders and fitness models widely used this, it was later discovered that this was not only helping them lose body fat, but we're giving them better health benefits. People who followed the Warrior died not only did they lose body fat, but they noticed that their growth hormone and testosterone levels went up more specifically, they started to digest food a lot better. The reason why they were digesting food a lot better is that intermittent fasting was helping them to get rid of any toxins and to help them to become insulin sensitive.

As you know, when it comes to bettering your health, it is essential for you to see amazing results in the detoxification department. Intermittent fasting truly helped people get rid of any toxins in their system, whether it be debris or something more profound. The great thing about intermittent fasting is that it not only cleans you internally and through your stomach. What I mean by that is intermittent fasting detoxify you in many ways I can't even think about. This is where autophagy comes in, autophagy has shown to not only proved to detoxify your body, but it helps you with getting rid of any dead cells and replace it with new ones. There are many different ways to go about intermittent fasting; we will talk about those methods later on in this book. That being said, Intermittent fasting is a simple way of saying that you will be cyclically eating food. Some hours of the day, you will be fasting and only drinking water, whereas, on the other hours, you will be consuming food.

Autophagy

The body goes through a lot of metabolic processes. As a result, cells (or some of their parts) get damaged. This is normal. Some factors like aging, stress, and the onslaught of free radicals can result in even more considerable damage. Senescent cells are cells that remain in the organs and tissues but serve no real purpose. When damaged and senescent cells stay in the body, they tend to activate inflammatory pathways. Your immune system becomes weaker. You become an easy target for a wide range of diseases. Autophagy is a process that helps the body get rid of damaged and senescent cells. The word "autophagy" is a combination of the Greek words "auto'" which means self, and "phagy," which means eating. It refers to the body's natural metabolic process of eating its tissue, especially when the body is starved or ill. Autophagy is a survival mechanism. It is the body's way of responding to stress and protecting itself. In recent years, researchers have discovered that autophagy can prevent the early signs of aging. It appears to also have a wide range of benefits for the immune system, the nervous system, the cardiovascular system, and metabolism in general. By "eating itself," the body promotes the renewal of healthy cells. It destroys and eliminates damaged components found inside cells. It reuses the waste matter that cells produce and builds new material for the repair and regeneration of new cells. Autophagy helps the body "clean up." It makes the body stronger. It enables the body to fight stress and diseases. What Are the Benefits of Autophagy? Put, autophagy promotes health at the cellular level. It is a mechanism for health and self-preservation. It helps the body to clean, recycle, and regenerate new and healthy cells so that the body regains optimal function.

Here's a quick rundown of what autophagy does for the body:

- Autophagy provides energy and molecular building blocks for cells.

- It helps recycle damaged proteins and other cell tissues to rebuild the cells.

- It allows cells to produce usable energy from oxygen and nutrients.

- It helps the cells eliminate toxic substances.

- It makes DNA more stable.

- It keeps organs and tissues healthy by protecting the healthy cells and getting rid of harmful or diseased ones

- It has the potential for preventing or delaying neurodegenerative illnesses like Alzheimer's disease.

- It protects the nervous system and improves cognitive function by promoting the growth of healthy nerve cells.

- It protects the body from heart disease.

- It helps the immune system function more efficiently.

- It reduces inflammation

- It slows down aging.

- It helps with digestive health.

- It prevents cancer.

- It helps you manage your weight.

- It helps prevent heart disease, liver problems, diabetes, cancer, and other chronic health problems.

What Can You Do to Stimulate Autophagy?

All cells go through natural autophagy. They tend to go through more actively when they are under stress or become deprived of nutrients. You can induce autophagy. You can increase the stressors. You can also deliberately do things to deprive the body of nutrients. Physical exercise is a "good stressor." Fasting, on the other hand, is a temporary way to restrict calories and deprive the body of nutrients. Both have been identified as effective strategies for inducing autophagy. It is interesting to note that both exercise and calorie-restriction are approaches often recommended to control weight, delay aging, and inhibit a variety of age-associated illnesses.

1. Practice Fasting There is several things you can do to induce autophagy. Foremost among them is changing lifestyle habits and going on a diet. Studies show that the best thing you can do is to go on a fast. There is nothing complicated about fasting. You stop eating (or severely limit your food intake) for a specified period. You go without food, although you can still take water, tea, or coffee. IMF or Intermittent Fasting is a dietary strategy that has become quite popular. It generates serious interest because people who practice it seem to

enjoy many health benefits as a result of the diet. Here is a quick look at how fasting works: Intermittent fasting is a strategy where you eat only during specific periods. You have several options about how to do this. You can practice alternate-day fasting. On a fasting day, you limit yourself to having 1 or 2 meals that only contain around 500 calories. This will severely cut down the number of calories you take in. On a non-fasting day, you do not set any limit to what you eat. This means that you eat one day and fast the next day. You can also set an "eating window." You limit your eating to 4 to 8 hours and fast for the other 16 to 20 hours. What form of fasting works best for autophagy? Health care experts say that fasting between 24 to 48 hours can give you the most reliable results. However, most people find it challenging to go without food for such a relatively long period. A more comfortable option is to go without eating for between 12 and 36 hours at a time. You abstain from eating in between meals and stick to 1 or 2 nutrient-dense snacks a day. Have your last lunch between 6 and 7 at night and break your fast at 7 in the morning. If you can manage it, skip breakfast and have brunch between 11 and 12 noon. This schedule extends your fasting period and brings faster results. Once your stomach gets used to going without meals, you can go on occasional 2-to-3 day fasts.

2. Go on a Keto Diet Ketosis is a metabolic state characterized by the production of ketones. Ketosis is excellent for losing weight. It gives your body a stable supply of energy. You'll have greater focus and concentration. It produces a feeling of satiety that results in fewer hunger pangs and food cravings. The fastest way to achieve ketosis is by not eating anything (or going on a fast). A more natural way to achieve ketosis is to go on a keto diet. The keto or ketogenic diet brings results similar to those that you get from fasting. It is a low-carb, high-fat diet. You eat a lot of rich and fatty food and restrict your intake of carbohydrates. When you go on a ketogenic diet, you choose your food carefully. 75% of your daily calories should come from fat, and only 5 to 10% should come from carbohydrates. A keto diet includes substantial amounts of olive oil, high-fat coconut oil, butter, ghee (a semi-fluid clarified butter popular in South Asian cooking), fermented cheese, meat, seeds, nuts, and avocado. It also includes fiber-rich vegetables so you can fill your requirements for antioxidants and vitamins. Usually, your body gets its energy from glucose, a form of sugar that comes from carbohydrates. When there isn't enough glucose

available, the body turns to fat for fuel. The ketogenic diet gets its name from the word "keto." This is because the food makes the body produce ketones – small molecules that are used for fuel. Ketones are an alternative source of energy.

When the body uses up its supply of glucose (which is its principal source of energy), it turns to ketones to provide the fuel. The body produces ketones on a ketogenic diet. The diet includes a minimal amount of carbohydrates, protein in moderation, and a high degree of fatty food. The liver uses fat to produce ketones. When you go on a keto diet, your body switches from glucose to fat as its fuel source. It burns fat the entire time. When insulin levels decrease, the body burns fat faster. It turns to stored fat and burns them off.

What to Eat and Avoid on a Ketogenic Diet What to Eat A ketogenic nutritional plan is built around the following foods:

- Mackerel tuna, trout, salmon, and other fatty fish
- Turkey, chicken, ham, bacon, sausage, steak, and other red meat
- Omega 3 whole eggs or pastured eggs
- Grass-fed cream and butter

- Almonds, flax seeds, walnuts, chia seeds, pumpkin seeds, and other seeds and nuts

- Avocado oil, coconut oil, olive oil (preferably extra virgin), and other healthy oils

- Mozzarella, blue, goat, cheddar, cream, and other unprocessed cheese

- Guacamole, preferably freshly made, and whole avocados

- Peppers, onions, tomatoes, green leafy vegetables, and other low-carb veggies

- Spices, pepper, salt, healthy herbs, and other similar condiments What to Avoid Limit foods that are high in carbs. Reduce your intake of (or eliminate) the following foods from your diet:

- Candy, cake, ice-cream, fruit juice, soda, and other sugary foods

- Cereal, pasta, rice, wheat-based products, and other starches or grains

- Parsnips, carrots, sweet potatoes, potatoes, and other tubers and root vegetables

- All fruit except strawberries and other berries (but only in tiny portions)

- Chickpeas, lentils, kidney beans, peas, and other legumes or beans

- Diet products and other low-fat products which are usually carbs-rich and highly processed

- Sauces or condiments that are sweet

- Mayonnaise, highly processed vegetable oils and other unhealthy fats

- Alcoholic beverages (because of their high carb content)

3. Get Regular Physical Exercise Physical exercise is recognized as a good stressor. It induces autophagy, especially in the pancreas, liver, muscles, adipose tissues, and other organs involved in the regulation of metabolism. Exercise helps break down tissues and repair and regenerate them. Is it all right to exercise while you are fasting? Doing this may take some getting used to, especially when you haven't applied for a long time. Once you get used to fasting and see the results, however, you may even feel more motivated to exercise. While all forms of exercise induce autophagy, experts suggest that you include a few minutes of intense aerobic exercise in your program. Half an hour of intense cardiovascular exercise can cause autophagy in the

heart and skeletal muscle tissues. High-Intensity Interval Training or HIIT appears to be the best form of exercise to induce autophagy. It brings you to a sweet spot for good stress. It applies the right degree of importance to elicit biochemical change. HIIT is built around the short-term high-level stress concept. Using a HIIT exercise program (resistance training and weightlifting) for 30 minutes every other day helps you give autophagy a healthy boost. You can use the same concept for other forms of exercise. If you are fond of walking, you can alternate brisk walking and slower-paced walking to achieve similar results.

4. Get enough sleep.

Sleep has therapeutic benefits. If you sleep better, you tend to look younger, feel more energetic, and live longer. Your circadian rhythm (or your daily wake/sleep cycles) affects autophagy. If you can get quality rest and sleep, you trigger autophagy. You help activate your body's natural recycling program.

On the other hand, when you disturb your circadian rhythm, you also disrupt autophagy. When you get too much exposure to blue light from screens, you disturb your circadian rhythm. When you do not keep a regular and consistent schedule of sleeping and waking times, you disrupt your circadian rhythm. Sleep affects your physical and emotional well-being. It affects your waking life and can significantly diminish or enhance its quality. If you do not get the right amount of high-quality sleep, you feel its toll on your emotional balance, productivity, energy, and even your weight. You do not have to struggle or toss and turn for countless hours before you can fall asleep. You have to develop the right habits (affecting both your daytime and bedtime routine), so you can sleep better. Getting the right amount of sleep gives you a lot of health benefits. You become sharp and alert. You are more focused.

You have more energy. You can keep your emotions on an even keel. Some simple tips for better sleep include the following:

- Maintain a regular sleeping and waking schedule.
- Get enough sunlight.
- Get enough exercise during the day.
- Limit nicotine and caffeine.
- Avoid sugary snacks, especially at night.
- Do not overeat at dinner.

- Indulge in a warm bath.

- Turn off all technological gadgets 1 or 2 hours before sleep.

- Avoid blue screens an hour or two before your bedtime.

- Dim the lights in your bedroom just before turning in.

- Bring your bedroom's temperature down to 65 degrees.

- Use a sleep app or a sound machine to help you sleep better.

- Wind down through mediation or deep-breathing exercises before sleep.

Chapter 2: Benefits of Autophagy

Speaking of autophagy, there are a lot of benefits that come along with this process. What we will do in this chapter is to go through all the top health benefits that will come along once you achieve autophagy. The great thing about autophagy is that it helps you tremendously when it comes to detoxifying your body. Understanding that the main benefit behind autophagy is that it helps you to not only put on muscle and lose fat but, more specifically, helps you with detoxifying your body. The main premise behind autophagy is to help you detoxify; understanding this concept is very important. Also, consider the fact that most of the benefits that you will be seen from autophagy might be a placebo effect. You have to realize that most of the claims and benefits have not been backed by science, some of them are, but most of them haven't been backed up. With that being said, let's talk about the first benefit that you will see following autophagy.

Homeostasis

As you might know, are saggy helps you with achieving homeostasis. when you are practicing intermittent fasting is looking to achieve autophagy, you slow down the process of Aging. The reason why you will slow that down is that your body will be in homeostasis. Homeostasis is simply a position in your body where it feels very comfortable and healthy. There's not a lot of pressure on the body. Therefore, it can relax and stop fighting off any issues that they might be facing. To put it in simple terms, homeostasis is where you want to be if you are looking to stay healthy for a long time. Many studies suggest that homeostasis can be achieved using autophagy within eight weeks of following it. Many participants are followed by 16/8 intermittent fasting to shave their goal of homeostasis. Within eight weeks of following the intermittent fasting and some other practices, they noticed that their homeless cases were a lot more consistent, and they saw consistent results when it comes to putting on muscle, losing fat, and feeling good overall. All in all, achieving homeostasis will do you good, so make sure you try and be in this state.

Better Skin

As you know, autophagy helps you with detoxifying yourselves. The way detoxifies your body is by killing any dead cells that are present. This is one of the best ways to detoxify yourself, both internally and externally.

Moreover, what does detoxifying does for you is that it gets rid of any bad cells that you might have or what might be causing any issues. When you are getting rid of these dead cells, you are also better in your skin. Believe it or not, most of the time, people have lousy skin simply because of inflammation and improper detoxification.

As you know, autophagy is one of the best ways to detoxify your body, which is why I work so well when it comes to better in your skin. If you want better glowing skin, then we highly recommend that you follow intermittent fasting to achieve autophagy. There are many other ways to make autophagy. However, we recommend intermittent fasting as it has been proven to deliver. Keeping that in mind, if you have been noticing your skin getting worse by the day, then consider autophagy to change that up for you. Many people who are achieving autophagy have seen that their skin got a lot better, and they're looking a lot younger.

Sense of Well-being

Another thing autophagy can help you with is a sense of well-being. Now, this might sound confusing to you, but it is, in fact, a benefit, how to say you will help you feel a lot better about yourself answer grow as a person. The reason why helps you with a sense of well-being is that you will have an elevated mood when you are detoxified and Feeling Good by yourself internally and externally, you will feel useful in general. This is why autophagy works so well when it comes to making you healthy overall since it helps you to feel a lot better about yourself when you detoxify yourself. More specifically, if you are following intermittent fasting, then chances are you will have a lot less mental fog as it has been proven scientifically to do so. So if you are someone looking to feel better by yourself throughout the day and have a sustained amount of dopamine level in your brain, then it is highly suggested that you started following intermittent fasting and to achieve autophagy. There have been studies showing that people who follow intermittent fasting to make autophagy increase their sense of well-being significantly. There have been many studies proving that, so if you have a problem with feeling good about yourself, then consider autophagy and intermittent fasting. Not to take this even more in-depth, autophagy has been shown scientifically to get rid of any old brain cells that you might have. When you are recycling your old brain cells and replacing them with new ones, you will notice a better sense of well-being and overall greatness. This is why many people who are very successful in their field tend to follow intermittent fasting and also feel good about themselves overall. If you are trying to be successful in any area, it is essential to have a sense of well-being and feeling good.

Cleanses Your Body

You already had an idea that we are going to be talking about this, but as you know, autophagy has been shown to cleanse your body internally and externally. Many people have an insane amount of inflammation in their skin, such as cyst or pimples. It is caused by dead cell collecting. I know we talked about skin health previously, but that was to talk about skin aging and wrinkles. Having pimples and cysts can, in fact, be a disease that could spread, which is why it has a section of its own. What autophagy does is clean your body internally and externally from any dead cells? When you are cleaning out your dead cells, you are also cleaning out any disease cells that you might have present in your body. This is why it is imperative to follow autophagy if you are looking to get rid of any issues that you might be facing when it comes to cysts and pimples. Also, when it comes to cleaning your body, autophagy has been shown to clean out your digestive system of any leftover matter. Unfortunately, in the United States, our colon is very coddled. And many people do not know how to get that fixed, one of the best ways to get that fix would be the following autophagy has it helps you to get rid of any intestine waste that you might have leftover. I know it sounds disgusting, but the truth is many people have leaky gut and fecal matter left in their bodies. One of the best ways to get rid of that is through Auto faking as you will be detoxifying your body internally and externally. If you do not know the ramifications of having feces left in your system, then you should know that it can be very toxic and can lead to illnesses in the future. Regardless if you follow autophagy or not, it is essential that you detoxify yourself regularly to upkeep with your health.

Cancer

As you know, autophagy has been shown to reduce the risk of cancer. If you do not know what cancer is, it is virtually cells that will not stop growing in your body and eating you to put it in simple terms. Now you know what I do not think he does, so you can see how it can help you with getting rid of cancer. Now I do not want to go on a limb here, but there have been many studies showing the autophagy is one of the best ways to get rid of cancer. When you start following intermittent fasting or any other diet which facilitates Auto Peggy, you will notice that you are detoxifying yourself very thoroughly. This is why you must follow autophagy if you want to reduce the risk of any diseases.

But as you know, cancer is one of the deadliest diseases anybody can have, so it is always good to be prepared when it comes to reducing the risk of any of these fatal diseases. The way autophagy works when it comes to reducing the risk of cancer is simply by killing off any dead cells that you might have present in your body. Once the body kills up any dead cells present in your body, the chances of cancer growth go to almost zero. As you know, chemotherapy does the same thing, but you pay tens of thousands of dollars for it. So my advice to you would be not to spend that much money and follow intermittent fasting to achieve autophagy.

Increase Hearth Health

There has been growing research showing that autophagy and intermittent fasting can help you get rid of any heart-related issues and diseases. When you are following intermittent fasting are looking to achieve autophagy, you will notice that your heart health will get a lot better if you take care of your system. The way autophagy works when it comes to bettering your heart health is by reducing cholesterol. There have been numerous amounts of research showing that autophagy can help you with heart health by merely lowering your harmful cholesterol levels. This is why it is highly recommended to practice intermittent fasting if you are someone looking to better yourself with better eating habits. Now keep in mind that most of this research has not been proven, which is why whatever you read about autophagy and increase heart health take it with a grain of salt. With that being said, there have been many claims adjusting the Auto Peggy has helped people reduce the risk of heart diseases. It is easy to believe as autophagy does lower your cholesterol levels; however, it has never been linked to lowering heart diseases.

Inflammation

As you know, intermittent fasting has been proven to reduce inflammation. However, when following autophagy, you will reduce your inflammation tremendously. You might have heard about the anti-inflammatory diet. However, it's merely telling you to eat food which is low in acidic level. What is the figure does makes it very easy for you to not only lower the risk of inflammation but the help you stay relatively free. What I mean by free is that you will not be restricted by the foods that you can and cannot eat.

Moreover, the information will be decreased because when you are following autophagy, you are detoxifying yourself when you are detoxing yourself, you are getting rid of dead cells, which can cause inflammation. Inflammation is simply the body's response to injury. Most of the time, these injuries are caused by not detoxifying yourself on time. That being said, reducing inflammation can help you out regardless of what you think, which is why you need to understand this issue of inflammation and how to get rid of it appropriately. The truth is, many people have to take medications for their inflammation, and that is fine, as long as you are consulting your doctor. However, if you have any sign of inflammation, then intermittent fasting and autophagy can help you tremendously when it comes to getting rid of it. So make sure that you follow intermittent fasting and autophagy to reduce information, as a truly will change your overall sense of well-being and inflammation.

Hormone Imbalance

We live in a society where hormone imbalances are a norm, which is not a good thing as hormone imbalances can cause many issues. What autophagy does that help you to balance out all your hormones, so you are in a good place? Believe it or not, hormones can make a big difference in how you react to things and how your body functions. For example, if you have a lot of estrogen in your body and you are a male, you will start behaving like a female figuratively speaking. However, hormones can make a drastic change in how you act. Keeping that in mind, what intermittent fasting and autophagy do is that not only increases the hormones that your body needs, but it also helps you with balancing them out, so you do not have any issues with them. If you do not know, intermittent fasting has been shown to increase your growth hormone level. Which is a good thing as that can lead to numerous amounts of health benefits. That being said, when following intermittent fasting and achieving autophagy, you will see vast numbers of benefits when it comes to fixing any hormone imbalances which you might be facing.

Enhances the Immune System

As you are well aware of this benefit, having a sound immune system can do tremendous things to you. Not only does having a sound immune system help you with reducing common cold and flu symptoms, but it also helps you to live a longer life overall. As you know, detoxifying your body can increase immune system health. This is why we recommend you follow intermittent fasting and autophagy to achieve a better immune system. There have been many studies showing that people who follow intermittent fasting tend to get sick a lot less than people who do not. This is directly linked to better immune system health, so if you are someone who has a weak immune system, then chances are intermittent fasting. Autophagy can help you tremendously when it comes to bettering or strengthening that for you. More specifically, if you are someone who gets sick very often, then enhancing your immune system is something you need for longevity and overall wellness.

Weight Loss

If you are following intermittent fasting, the chances are that you will be losing a lot of weight and achieving autophagy at the same time. The reason why it works so well is that intermittent fasting not only burns fat for energy, but it also helps you with achieving autophagy. So when you are looking to meet autophagy, you will notice a substantial amount of weight loss. This is one of the best benefits when it comes to the following autophagy not only will you see tremendous amounts of health benefits, but you will also notice that you are losing weight. Many people start following diets to look better, so if you are someone who's looking to look a lot better, then you need to look into intermittent fasting and autophagy. There have been numerous studies showing the artifact he can help you reduce body fat tremendously. Most of the time, people are looking to lose weight, but they should be focusing on losing body fat. The last thing I want to do is lose muscle mass, as muscle mass can be right for you. However, when you are following autophagy, you will be explicitly losing fat, which can be one of the best benefits when it comes to monitoring intermittent fasting and autophagy.

Muscle Gain

As you remember, we talked about losing body fat; however, autophagy and intermittent fasting can help you put on muscle tremendously as well. We talked about hormones and how important they are when it comes to overall wellness and well-being. The great news about following Auto Peggy and looking towards achieving that is that it helps you balance out your hormones, which will, therefore, help you to put on a lot more muscle. Many athletes follow intermittent fasting and autophagy to better their athletic performance and to put on muscle. Now, if you are someone whose goal is to put on muscle, naturally than autophagy and intermittent fasting is the answer for you. For many people, this method might sound unorthodox when it comes to putting on muscle, but believe it or not, this is one of the best ways to put on natural muscle athletes.

To close off this chapter, we would like to remind you that autophagy and intermittent fasting is one of the best ways to achieve success with your health. We spoke about many benefits that come along with autophagy and intermittent fasting, and by the benefits research, you can tell that this is one of the best ways to go about achieving overall health and wellness. So if you are someone who's looking to change their body and mental capacity completely, then this is one of the best diets to follow. Keep in mind up intermittent fasting might not be the right solution for you if you have some health issues, so make sure they consult with your doctor before you follow any of these diet plans. Nonetheless, if you are a healthy person who's looking to see amazing results, then autophagy and intermittent fasting can be one of the best ways to go about achieving your goals.

Chapter 3: How Can Autophagy Get Rid of Diseases

There have been many studies showings that autophagy can help with reducing the risk of cancer, which is why this diet is one of the best things to follow when it comes to reducing the risk of any disease that you might be facing. Many studies are showing that most people who have cancer and started following autophagy fought off cancer and started to live a healthy life. Which is why we always recommend that you follow the autophagy when it comes to reducing the risk of cancer, or if you already have cancer, you can follow this diet to get rid of it. However, if you are facing cancer, then make sure to consult your doctor before you make any abrupt decisions.

The reason why autophagy works so well when it comes to reducing the risk of cancer is that it lowers your acidic level. When you have lower acidic levels, there's less chance of your body attracting more foul bacteria in your body, which will cause cancer. This environment will discourage any cancer surviving growth, which is why many people recommend you follow autophagy. Some people might say autophagy is not the right answer when it comes to reducing the risk of cancer; in fact, most people said as long as you eat healthy foods, then you will reduce the risk of cancer. However, many studies are showing that your lung and your other organs might be higher in the acidic level, which is why you are attracting more cancer in your body. The main thing you need to understand when it comes to reducing the risk of cancer is that cancer likes to thrive on acidic levels.

If your body is very acidic, you will be at a higher risk of attracting cancer regardless, which is why autophagy works so well at reducing the risk of cancer. Moreover, people have also shown to reduce the risk of inflammation, which makes it a great idea to follow autophagy when it comes to reducing the risk of cancer. As you might or might not know, one of the main reasons why we attract disease is the inflammation in our body. Many people get cancer because they are inflamed, and it's causing issues overall, increasing the risk of cancer.

Once people start losing the inflammation in the body, the risk of cancer lowers even further, making it a great idea to start following autophagy as autophagy reduces the risk of cancer and inflammation in your body. Also, as you know, autophagy has shown to rejuvenate our body. Once you start to break down your old cells and come out with new ones, your body will have more fighting power towards the cancerous cells.

You are making the autophagy one of the best diets to follow when it comes to reducing the risk of cancer. If your goal is to live a healthier life, then one of the main things you need to understand is your body recycling and detoxifying it very quickly. This is where the autophagy comes on. Any time you detoxify your body will be in much better shape to get rid of any diseases, more specifically cancer. Anyhow, many people go on fasts and other things to detoxify the body. This can also come in handy when it comes to reducing the risk of cancer, but the way these diet works is so correctly that does not only detoxify your body but also makes it an autophagy environment where bacteria, which because cancer cannot survive. Also, when you are eating these high autophagy foods, you are not only making it better for yourself to reduce the risk of cancer. You are also making your body more bacteria-friendly, as you will be adding more good bacteria in your body, helping you fight off the harmful bacteria in your body. As you might know, we have two types of bacteria in our body, and we have the good ones and the bad ones. We ideally want good bacteria in your body to fight off any disease that we might notice. Which means you need to make sure that you have good bacteria in your diet. As you know, autophagy provides you with good bacteria and lots of it. However, it would be best if you made sure that when you have these good bacteria is in your body that you are drinking enough water to digest it and to keep your gut healthy.

This is why you must drink more water, which we will talk about that later in this book. However, for now, you need to understand the importance of good bacteria in your body and reducing cancer, overall if your goals to minimize cancer autophagy will provide you with that. However, if your goal is to reap all the benefits from the autophagy, then you need to make sure that a couple of things are in check before you do so. You need to make sure they get an ample amount of protein, fats, and carbs in your diet. As your diet will be very restricted when it comes to the food you are going to be eating, you need to make sure that you are eating the right macronutrients for your body. This means we need to make sure that you are eating foods that will give you a balanced macronutrient breakdown.

You will be eating no meat, which means you'll have to make up your protein needs are met through plant-based meals and plant-based products. We will give you some fantastic recipes to make good food. However, your goal is to understand that you are hitting the right number of calories for your required body fat on your goals. If you are not eating an ample amount of food, then your body will not have enough energy to fight off these diseases or problems. Which is why you need to understand how many calories you need and eat accordingly based on that. Some people are claiming that you need to be eating enough food regardless of how much or what type of food intake you are following, which means that it is more recommended that you eat enough food to get the optimal results. If you are going through chemotherapy, then you need to be making sure they are eating enough food regardless of what diet you are following. If you want to make sure that your chemotherapy goes successful, then you must maintain your weight when you are going through this procedure.

There are some claims made that the autophagy will make it more successful for you when it comes to achieving chemotherapy success. However, many people are claiming this is entirely bogus. No claims are backing up that autophagy helps with chemotherapy.

However, many applications are suggesting that the autophagy will help you with reducing the risk of cancer and are getting rid of cancer entirely if you are following the diet. If you talk to your doctor, he or she will tell you that autophagy is one of the best diets to follow when it comes to reducing the risk of cancer. However, this is not the popular answer for most people.

As many people have been brainwashed with media saying that autophagy is not the best way to go about, if the professionals are saying that the autophagy is a great idea, there's some truth behind that. To clarify, there have not been many studies claiming that the autophagy will ultimately help you get rid of cancer. Nonetheless, there have been many real-life situations where this diet has helped.

If you want to make sure that you are getting the best results possible, then make sure that you combine it with a tasty smoothie routine, which will allow you to detoxify your body. It does not matter what diet you follow. If you aren't monitoring the autophagy or your organization is alkaline, then there's a high chance that you will not reduce the risk of cancer. Which means you will be in a much better position following the autophagy when it comes to reducing the risk of cancer, many professionals have claimed as such. One more thing to remember, if you are on acidic medications then you can counteract that with autophagy. Make sure that the medicines that you are taking aren't going to disrupt your autophagy. We can't tell you which medicine will cause you to be acidic, the best way to understand which ones will is to ask your doctor.

To recap, the autophagy will help you keep your body at an autophagy level, which will allow no cancer or bacteria to start activating or to start forming. The autophagy will detoxify you and create new cells which will enable you to fight off disease and make your immune system even stronger. Moreover, autophagy will also help you with chemotherapy, as many people have said it will. They are making this diet a no-brainer to follow. Just make sure that you are eating enough calories to maintain your body weight, especially if you are facing any cancerous diseases. I hope you understand how following autophagy can help you with reducing the risk of cancer and many other conditions, to clarify, there have been no studies showing that autophagy will help you to get rid of cancer or any different sorts of diseases.

This has been a personal recommendation of many doctors and an own review of many patients that autophagy has helped them tremendously to reduce the risk of cancer or many other diseases, which does make sense when you look at the benefits of autophagy. If you are facing any of these diseases, then always consult with your doctor before you start any of this diet. Moreover, as always, know what type of medications you are taking and how you can counterbalance your autophagy. Finally, truly understand what the autophagy is if you have to read this book a couple of times if you are feeling lost.

If you were going to follow this diet blindly, then it would be like riding a bicycle without training wheels. You need to understand the diet before you start following it, and feel it out before you can commit to it. If you can commit to this diet, then you will be in a great position in terms of seeing the benefits. One of the only problems with this diet would be the precise requirements. Also, you cannot drink alcohol or take any particular types of medication when following the autophagy. Make sure they have everything checked before you proceed to follow this diet. Once you have managed to do that, then you will be in a perfect position to start following this diet and to see the benefits of it.

The Difference Between the pH Levels

Once you have started to follow the autophagy, you will notice that many people who do follow the autophagy tend to look at their urine samples and the saliva samples to find out their pH levels. As you know, many people who are following the autophagy need to make sure that their body is not acidic. This means they have to make sure that they are at an autophagy state by using urine or other bodily fluids to figure out how acidic or autophagy they are. In the previous chapter, we talked about 6.5, and 7.5 is the right amount to be in when it comes to pH level. That being said, there are tons of ways to test your pH levels. The main two are the saliva pH and the urine pH. Many people do not know this, but these two tests are very different. One will be a lot more acidic, where is the other one will not be as acidic when compared, which is why you must understand the difference between the two methods and how you should use them accordingly based on your goals. The first thing you need to know when it comes to pH levels is that the saliva will always be higher at the autophagy level. Depending on your diet, your saliva will be more readily available to see where your pH level is at.

This will factor in the food you have eaten and how you have digested the food. One of the things you need to keep in mind when checking your saliva is that if you have eaten anything which is very Alkaline, if so, then it will show that your body is an autophagy state, even if it isn't. This could be misleading over time, which is why many people recommend that you test your pH level when using the saliva test post 30 to 40 minutes of eating. Most of the time, your saliva will be the most accurate test. Unlike your urine, your urine will be a lot more acidic nature and will be less autophagy when it comes to testing the autophagy level. There's a reason to that, the main reason why the autophagy level will be a lot lower in the urine is for a straightforward reason, which is that your urine normally gets rid of toxins in your body. Especially in the morning when you wake up, and you haven't urinated in a long time, your body will be cleaning out all your organs and pissing out all the bad things that are available in your body, which is why your urine will always be a lot more acidic when compared to your spit or saliva. Now when people are following autophagy, most of the time, they test both the urine level pH and their saliva level pH to get a better understanding of their body. You have to understand, when you are urinating, you are getting rid of toxins, which are, most of the time, very acidic.

Which is why you need to understand how to read your urine samples accordingly, your urine also contains a lot of sodium and waste products from all your organs, which is why specialist measure the pH level differently. The average pH level in urine is 6 pH; anything under 5 will be considered acidic. However, anything higher than 8 is alkaline. The same thing when it comes to saliva pH levels, your level will fluctuate on how much food you are eating and what kind of foods are going to be eating. For example, a high protein meal before you test your pH level using the urine test will lead to a higher acidic level, which is why we recommend you wait it out. However, if you have a high autophagy level in your urine, there's a high chance that you might have thrown up a lot, or you might have urinary tract infection. It is not ideal to be highly autophagy when it comes to following this diet. However, it can cause a lot of issues once you start monitoring this autophagy if you do not balance it up properly. You have to understand that you cannot be overly acidic or overly alkaline. Ideally, you want to be more on the autophagy side, which is why you need to be eating more autophagy foods to see better results, as previously mentioned. However, your urine will always be on the acidic side, so be aware of that once you start following this diet. The water you drink is also going to dictate how acidic you are once you start following this diet.

Also, the pH level in the urine can vary differently. Many doctors do not even use urine pH level test anymore as it is so unreliable. The doctor will only use the urine pH level to understand more information if needed. Many doctors will not even use the urine pH levels anymore, which is why we recommend that you do not use it either. However, if you are still stern about using this method, then there's a specific kit you can get at the drugstore, which will let you urinate in a box and will test out your pH level accordingly. Since there a lot of methods to test it out, we're not going to get into all the methods of testing out your urine samples and your pH levels. Just make sure that you go to the drug store and figure out which one you want to go with, and then use it accordingly.

This is if you want to test your pH level using the urine samples, if you are eating a right amount of autophagy food then there are no worries when it comes to testing out urine levels and your pH levels overall. On the other hand, the spit or saliva pH level can be beneficial. When it comes to testing out your saliva levels of pH level, you must understand how to use it properly and how to get the best results out of it. You have to realize that the saliva level will be a lot more accurate when it comes to testing out your pH level. As we told you previously, saliva does not hold any of the toxicity which urine does. Most of the time, saliva gives you a better understanding of where your pH level is throughout the whole diet.

Your pH level should be around 6 to 8 when you are testing out your saliva levels. Ideally, your pH level should be at 7.5, as this will give you the best results. This is one of the best areas to be in when it comes to being alkaline. To test out your saliva level, it is very straightforward, go to your nearest drug store and get those strips that will allow you to get your pH level reading. The first thing you need to do is take the colored part on top off the piece and put it underneath your tongue, making sure you get enough saliva on it. Once you've gotten enough saliva in the piece, then take it out after 30 seconds of putting it in your mouth and shake it up, it will give you a color scheme which will provide you with an idea where your pH level is. This is one of the best ways to test your pH level overall, this is very inexpensive and will give you a good idea of where your pH level is.

Just like the keto strips, you get online; it is similar to the keto strip. Instead, it will test out your pH levels. One thing to make sure when you start your test out your pH level using your saliva is to make sure that you haven't eaten or drunk any autophagy water before you test it. Give yourself at least 20 to 30 minutes before you start to use them autophagy strip to see where your pH level is, as we previously told you whatever you eat will show up on the pH test.

This is something you do not want; we want to understand where your pH level is naturally in our body and not by the foods that we just recently ate. We understand that the specific foods that we're going to be eating to alkalize your body are essential; however, once you do eat those autophagy foods, it will give you an unauthentic pH level reading. This sometimes happens after eating autophagy food, and your pH level tends to show up around 8 or 9, which is not an excellent spot to be in and can scare off more people. Make sure when you do test out your pH level that it is properly scheduled, and you haven't eaten in about 20 to 30 minutes, this will give you the best reading when it comes to pH level reading overall.

Now, the ideal urine and saliva pH sample should be around 7.2 when factored in both of their results. If you do both a urine sample and a saliva sample, and the average of both is 7.2 pH, then you are it the perfect spot. If your saliva sample goes below 7, then there's a high chance of your body starting to become acidic, which is what you need to understand, add more autophagy foods, which will allow you to become less acidic hence making you more alkaline. The recommended times you should be checking your pH level varies from person to person, and some people will say that you should check your pH level every two to three times a day.

However, some people recommend that you only need to check your pH level two to three times a week. We have found the best time which would be to test your pH level once a day, depending on how acidic or autophagy you are you might need to monitor it a little bit more. The best way to go about this would be to monitor it once a day. However, if you are more acidic and you are looking to become autophagy very quickly, then we recommend that you check your saliva pH level two to three times a day to see where your levels are at for a week or two. Once you've achieved a good level of pH levels, then it will be time to let it rest and then check your pH level less frequently these eating plans allowing you to save money on strips and have a better idea on where your pH levels are.

Once you become autophagy and your body becomes more alkalized, the chances of you finding out how acidic you are will drop. You see, when you are more alkaline, your insulin levels will drop, your inflammation levels will drop, and you will notice less pain overall. Once you become more acidic, your digestion will slow down, and you will feel more pain, and your inflammation will go up. These are a great sign to see when you are acidic or when you are alkaline. Understand your body is very important, which is why we highly recommend you start understanding how your body functions when it is acidic and when it is alkaline. As mentioned in the chapter, just so you can understand a little bit better, the first thing you need to do is understand that the urine sample is to be you are used on a rare occasion or if you want to be extra meticulous with your pH level. Many doctors do not even recommend that you use the pH level for urine to test out your pH level overall, as urine levels can be very unreliable when it comes to testing out your pH levels. Your saliva pH levels will be a lot more accurate for the average person to test on how acidic or autophagy you are. If you are to test your saliva and your urine pH levels, then make sure that your pH level is at 7.2, which will make it the ideal pH level overall when it comes to making sure that you are at the autophagy side of the body.

As always, when you are testing your urine pH level that you test it after you have done urinating first thing in the morning, ideally midday when you have drunk enough water and your liver and other organs have been cleaned up. On the other side your saliva test should not be done once you have eaten anything, ideally, wait for 30 to 40 minutes before you test your pH level after you are done eating food as this could give you a wrong reading once you have eaten a portion of food and test your pH level right after.

The foods can dictate how your pH levels going to be, which is why it is ideal that you wait down a bit before you test out your pH levels. Furthermore, depending on your acidic levels, you also need to understand how your body functions when it is a lot more acidic, and when it is more alkaline. That way, you do not have to keep testing your pH levels, and you can tell by the way your body is performing to get a better idea of your acidic or autophagy levels. If you do eat autophagy or acidic food, make sure to counteract it by eating a different type of food to make sure that your pH level is balanced. With that in mind, now you've got a good idea of how to test your pH levels and the different types of pH levels when it comes to you being autophagy and acidic overall. You can now utilize the right methods, which you think will benefit you greatly, after reading this chapter. Make sure that you do not spend too much money on pH level strips, as it is essential that you do not take this very seriously. In the beginning, it is ideal that you test your pH levels regularly. However, once you have gotten the idea of how your body feels when it is acidic or alkaline, then you will not have to check it so frequently.

Chapter 4: Which Fasting Protocol to Follow

As you know by now, intermittent fasting is perhaps the best way to achieve true autophagy. In this chapter, we will help you figure out which intermittent fasting plan you can follow. One of the great things about intermittent fasting would be that it goes by your lifestyle and needs and that it can be catered accordingly, which is what makes intermittent fasting so great and effective. With that in mind, let's talk about the ways you can achieve autophagy.

Pick the Right Plan

It is essential that you pick out the right fasting protocols for your needs. As you could tell, they were all different, but none the less effective in their manner. Every fasting approach tends to yield different types of results, so it is essential that you picked the right one, which works with your lifestyle and your goals. What we will do is go through all the fasting methods step by step and explain to you which one is suited for what type of goals and lifestyle, and after reading those, you can decide on which one to start following. If that sounds good, let's get started, we will begin by talking about the 12 hours fast.

12-hour fast: As we previously mentioned, 12 hours fast is for someone who is a beginner in the realm of intermittent fasting. It is best followed by people who are just trying to get their feet wet, the 12-hour fast works many different ways. The 12-hour fast will help you clean out your digestive system, and will also help with weight loss. This fasting protocol is very similar to the 16 hours fast, and sometimes known as the baby 16 hours fast because it is a stepping stone to other fasting methods. If your primary goal is to lose fat, and to see some significant benefits from fasting, then this would be ideal for you. This fast is very manageable in regards to setting time for eating and fasting window, and you can fit in this intermittent fasting method at any time there is no specific window, which makes this ideal for busybodies.

16-hour fast: Very similar to the 12-hour fast, the 16-hour fast is one of the most popular fasting methods used by many. This method is for people who are trying to lose weight, build muscle, and live an overall healthy life. If your goal is to get results from autophagy, then this fasting method might be for you, as this is one of the fasting protocols which have been proven to promote autophagy. This plan is perfect for people who are following the 12-hour fast and are looking for a bump, similar effects of the 12-hour fast. It is just prolonged for 4 hours. If you are someone looking to get the most of the health benefits from intermittent fasting, then this plan is for you. Moreover, if you are someone who demands flexibility with the eating windows, then this plan would be better suited for you.

Fast for two days per week: Also known as the 5:2 method, this is one of the more intense fasting protocols. Even though there have been zero studies showing the health benefits by following a 5:2 method, it is best known for drastic weight loss. If you are looking to lose weight quickly and efficiently, this plan might be the answer for you. One thing to remember this plan who's better suited for women who had some experience with intermittent fasting, do not start following this plan if you are a complete beginner. This plan can be straightforward to cope with on day to day basis, as you can merely fast when you are not working. Overall this plan is excellent for intermediate fasters who are looking to lose weight quickly, and one suggestion would be to not follow this plan for longer than four weeks.

Alternative day fasting: very similar to the 5:2 method, you fast for one day, and you usually eat the next day, so on and so forth. Most of the time, it works out be three days of fasting and four days off eating healthy. This method is a little bit more aggressive when it comes to weight loss, where the 5:2 approach puts you in a 20% calorie deficit for the whole week; this puts you in a 25% calorie deficit, making it an advanced protocol. If you are someone who has experienced intermittent fasting and are looking to lose weight quickly, then I would highly recommend this plan to you, as this is one of the most aggressive yet safe ways to lose body fat. However, again, make sure you follow it for less than four weeks.

Weekly 24-hour fast: It requires you to only fast once a week for 24 hours, quite frankly I'm not a fan of this fasting method, but I know many people use it. Some benefits are showing that it might help with cleaning out your gut, and helping you with overall weight loss as it will put you in a 5% caloric deficit for the week. This plan can be used by anyone, as you can fast on the days off. Overall I am not a fan of this fasting protocol, but it is there for you to follow.

Meal skipping: Meal skipping is one of the most natural fasting protocols out there, if you are a complete beginner who is very scared to start intermittent fasting then this might be the stepping stone for you. Even though there will be minimal benefits from this fasting protocols, it will teach beginners to listen to their body. Overall helping you understand how your body works when in starvation mode and help you show how to deal with hunger.

The warrior diet: The warrior diet, where you fast for 20 hours and eat for 4 hours. In the four hours, you are allowed to eat whatever you want, just like any fasting method. Ideally, this fasting method was made for people looking to lose weight and gain muscle, hence the name. However, this diet is no different from the 16 hours fast, and there are no added benefits to fasting for extra hours from 16 to 20. If you are someone looking to make you are fasting a bit more challenging or shorten your eating window to lower your caloric intake, then this plan can be for you. This plan can tire you out very quickly, from personal experience, if you have a lot going with your work-life, then stick with the 16 hours fast.

This information should help you tremendously with picking out the fasting protocol for your needs, make sure it is sustainable for you.

Macros Suggestion

Intermittent fasting works excellent, but it works a lot better when you eat healthier overall. For you to achieve better results from intermittent fasting, it needs to be health-focused meals. You see, when you start following intermittent fasting alongside a healthy diet, and magic starts to happen. What we will do is give you pointers on how to begin observing intermittent fasting the right way.

We previously method before the macros and the eating patterns we recommended for people intermittent fasting, so let us recap them. If your goal is to lose body fat your macros should be 40% protein 20% carbs and 40% fats, whereas if your goal is to maintain your weight and reap the benefits of intermittent fasting, then we recommend following a macro protocol of 30% protein 40% carbs and 30% fats. If you want to lose weight, then you need to look at your diet, making sure you do not go over your calories and macros. If you aren't eating healthy meals throughout the day, then you can slowly start to incorporate better meals.

Start by having one healthy meal when you break your fast and one meal of whatever you desire, and once you become more comfortable, you can make it two meals. Making you slowly start eating healthier, which will yield even better results overall. Yes, many people do get away with eating foods that aren't healthy, and yes, they so see unusual changes. However, if you want to see over the top changes, then we recommend eating a bit more robust. Now there is no specific diet you need to follow; merely make healthier choices as this should help. You need to take a look at your food which you are eating and make changes where necessary. It will be hard in the beginning, but it will eventually become more natural.

Be Careful

It's imperative that you listen to your body when you are fasting. Listening to your body will help you understand stop and will not stop. Intermittent fasting for women can require extra attention, and that is why it is necessary to listen to your body. There are some telltale signs to look out for when doing intermittent fasting, know that most of the symptoms should subside within a week.

However, if they do not, chances are you need to switch up your fasting protocol. One of the ways to tell the intermittent fasting is becoming way too hard for you, is when you start feeling cold chronically. Once you begin to feel cold chronically, that's a big sign that intermittent fasting is becoming very hard for you to follow if you feel cold throughout the day for three weeks plus then chances are it is time for you to lower the fasting intensity. Another sign to consider when you are intermittent fasting would be the extreme hunger.

In the first couple of weeks, you will feel extreme hunger, but if that keeps happening for over three weeks, chances are your body is telling you that you can't follow intermittent fasting at this level. These are the significant signs you need to listen to your body when intermittent fasting, but always make sure you get your blood work done and get the professional help if you feel like intermittent fasting is affecting you physically. Best rules to live by when intermittent fasting if it does not feel right three weeks into it then stop. Nonetheless, symptoms could occur anytime, be intuned with your body, and make sure you are listening to it.

How to Deal With Hunger

When following an intermittent fasting routine, it is crucial that you make sure that your appetite is under control to make sure fast isn't broken prematurely. Time and time again, many followers of the intermittent fasting have broken the fast prematurely just because they couldn't control their hunger. We will go multiple ways to deal with desire, and overall help you continue with intermittent fasting. The first tip is pretty obvious, and that is to drink more water. Much of the time, hunger is thirst.

Meaning you will be able to control your eating desires by drinking more water, having more water through the day helps you tremendously to control your hunger. Another method for managing your appetite would be to drink more coffee and green tea, and caffeine has shown to suppress, which overall helps you with fasting. Just make sure the coffee or tea you drink does not contain any sugar or milk, as that could break your fast. Getting yourself busy will help you control your hunger. Most of the time, when we occupy yourself with work, we tend to forget the food.

Perhaps do some work or household chores to keep yourself busy when you feel like eating. You can also exercise or go for a walk, and this will kill two birds with one stone. When you start walking, you will take your mind of fasting, and you will also burn some fat while doing so. If you are feeling more energetic, then you can go ahead and get a full workout. However, remember that you might feel hungry after the exercise if you have no experience in managing your hunger. Now, if you are looking for a more relaxed way of handling your appetite, then we would recommend meditation.

Meditation works well when it comes to controlling your hunger, and it will also help you manage your mental stress if you have any. Make sure you are using this tool to manage your appetite, and who knows you might enjoy meditation. The final technique we recommend would be to eat more fibrous foods before you start your fast, as this will help you stay fuller for an extended period. Many followers of intermittent fasting will eat junk food, and this will make them crave foods faster than someone who ate a good healthy meal with a ton of fiber in it.

If you want to have a better, less hungry fasting window, then we highly recommend you eat healthy meals with a ton of fiber in them before you start fasting. These are all the tips and tricks to dealing with hunger, make sure that you are following all these tips to control your appetite when fasting. Especially if it is your first three weeks fasting, as that is when you will notice most of the hunger cravings, these tips will help you tremendously to power through those first three weeks, and help you with completing your fast.

Progress Tracking

If you want to be successful with intermittent fasting, then you need to start tracking your progress. Tracking your progress is the main reason why most people continue with intermittent fasting and why most people do not, and there's a reason for that. You see, when you start tracking your daily progress, you will begin to notice better results, which will help you hold yourself accountable to it. There are three ways to track your progress when intermittent fasting, and we will talk about those today. The first way you can track your progress is by daily journaling, write down everything how you felt and how your body was feeling when fasting.

Not only will this teach you how to listen to your body, but it would also show your progress, so if you are ever feeling down, you can go back and read past experiences and results with intermittent fasting and see how much better you have gotten. Another method to track your fasting would be to schedule out your whole week in terms of time frame like when it comes to fasting and eating window. Most people go day-by-day fasting whenever they feel, which is fine, but you'll see much better results if you figure out your whole week, so set up your fasting windows and eating windows.

This method would also help you stay accountable for your fasting goals. The third way to track your progress would be to measure your body composition every week. This will not only keep you motivated in terms of keeping you moving forward, but it would also help you see how you are progressing, and if changes are needed to be made. These are the three main ways to track your progress and to stay on track with intermittent fasting, and we recommend using all three.

Remember that most people give up or quit because they do not have a plan or a strategy to get somewhere. Once you start tracking your progress and tracking your intermittent fasting schedules, you will notice that you are a lot more accountable with your goals, and you will begin to see better results.

We highly recommend you start tracking your progress and mainly use these tools that we just talked about. There are also apps that can be used to track your progress. If you do not like writing stuff out, then you can download apps that will help you to track your progress. Overall there should be no excuse not to track your progress. Also, we recommend you journal your body composition weekly and your journaling daily.

The journaling works a lot better when written daily since your emotions are at its peak when you write them out. However, if you feel that daily journaling can become hard, you can also journal weekly. Nonetheless, daily journaling is a lot better. Follow whatever feels best for you, but remember to track all three progress to see better results; it does not matter how you track it as long you monitor it.

Chapter 5: Who Can Fast?

While intermittent fast is flexible and does not restrict what you eat, if you want to lose weight and be healthy, you should ideally avoid junk foods. Sticking to a well-balanced and nutrient-rich diet will help you lose weight quickly and will also help you avoid many chronic and often fatal diseases and disorders. A well-balanced meal is necessary while fasting because it will keep you energized and fulfill your quota of essential nutrients for the day. If you continue to eat junk food in your eating period regularly, you will essentially undo whatever positive results you gain from fasting. All the hard work will go down the drain.

So, instead of consuming a lot of junk food, try to stick to a healthy and, if possible, low-carb foods as much as possible. This does not mean that you should not indulge in junk food once in a while. The best thing about intermittent fasting is that it focuses on when you eat and not on what you eat, so unlike other diets, you are allowed to eat junk food and other guilty pleasures whenever you want.

Just remember to avoid overdoing it. It is clear that intermittent fasting is a versatile form of diet that has multiple benefits. It is clear that there are many different things that you can do to get the best and most out of intermittent fasting. Yet, you should expect constant and rapid weight loss while doing the intermittent fast. You will see a heavyweight loss in the beginning. Your body will soon adapt to low calories, and you may stop losing for a while, but do not worry, this is a common peak and plateau situation, and you will soon start losing weight once again.

The effects of intermittent fasting are best noticed in the first few weeks, where many people report dramatic weight loss. Like every other diet, the intermittent fasting will have a weight loss plateau as well. It is an inherent part of the weight loss process that can neither be ignored nor can it be avoided. The only thing that can be done in such cases is to avoid getting frustrated and dejected and carry on the fast with added vigilance and focus. Try to keep consistent and avoid changing too much, and in a week or two, you will soon start noticing weight loss again. Keeping to the course will help you stay focused and will avoid disrupting the system too much. Stay focused and lose weight.

If you perform this diet properly, you will be able to reap all the benefits that are associated with this diet. This chapter will help to resolve all the confusion and problems that you may have about the intermittent fast. Who shouldn't fast? Intermittent fasting is one of the safest diets as it is backed by science, tradition, and history, so it is safe for almost everyone. It is an effective eating plan that focuses more on health and nutrition than other details. You get all the necessary calories and nutrients while doing this diet. Thus, it is safe for almost everyone. While almost everyone can do this diet, there are certain demographics who should avoid this diet or who should consult with their doctor before beginning this diet. It is possible that certain people will not be able to get enough nutrition from this diet, and it is recommended for such people to avoid this diet completely. For instance, if you are considered underweight or undernourished, you should avoid this diet completely. You should avoid any kind of diet completely unless specifically prescribed by a doctor. Fasting should be avoided by women who are pregnant and/or are breastfeeding. You are supposed to consume extra nutrients in pregnancy, or while you are breastfeeding, intermittent fasting will prove to be counterproductive to you. In some other cases, you are allowed to fast. You must check with your doctor first. This is the case with people who suffer from type 1 or Type 2 diabetes. Certain diabetes medicines can react negatively with fasts. If you have gout or high uric acid, you should avoid fasting, as well. Can fasting induce starvation mode? The simple answer to this question is yes and no. Intermittent fasting is shrouded with myths, and many times, these myths have been repeated as truths. Let us have a look at some of the most common myths associated with intermittent fasting.

- Fasting leads to starvation. (It may if you overdo it by a significant margin.)

- Fasting will leave you feeling uncomfortable and hungry.

- Fasting often leads to overeating. (It may happen in the beginning.)

- Fasting can make you lose muscle tone. All these myths have been disproved multiple times. Fasting does not lead to starvation; instead, the body will actually start burning extra fats stored in the body instead. Intermittent fasting is a great way to burn those stubborn fats stuck to your belly.

If you consume around 1000 meals a year for 50 years, you will consume a total of 50000 meals. Skipping some of these will not harm you in any way. Our body breaks muscle only when it has very low amounts of fats and when it does not get enough protein. If you face these two problems, then you should not fast anyway. Very few people actually have this issue because our body is made in such a way that it can go long without food. Are there any side effects of intermittent fast? There are certain side effects of fasting. They are either not so prominent or are rarely seen.

They are simple and often go away once your body becomes habitual of fasting. Let us have a look at some of the common side effects fasting. Constipation This is the most commonly seen side effect of fasting. If you are experiencing constipation, using natural laxatives like coffee can alleviate the pain quickly. Headaches Feeling lightheaded and headaches is another common problem associated with fasting. Once your body forms the habit of fasting, you will stop getting headaches. You can avoid headaches by consuming some extra salt with meals every day. Gurgling If you feel that your stomach is gurgling more than it normally does, you should drink mineral water instead of regular water for a few days.

Other Side effects: These may include dizziness, muscle cramps, heartburn, etc. Do not worry, though, these will go away on their own in a couple of days. How to Manage Hunger? Hunger may seem a bit difficult to manage in the beginning. You should understand that hunger would pass. Many people, while beginning the intermittent fast, believe that hunger will continue to grow, and soon you will not be able to tolerate it. This rarely happens.

Hunger does not build up; it comes in waves. To tackle hunger, you may drink lots of water, coffee, or tea to counter it. This will help you defeat hunger pangs. Extended fasts often lead to extra hunger. The hunger will increase the second day; however, after some time, you will see that hunger is receding. After three days, you will experience a complete loss of hunger. Here, your body will start using fats as a source of energy, which is why you will no longer feel hungry. In simple words, if you learn how to fast for a few days, your hunger pangs will disappear, and you will learn how to deal with hunger. You may struggle quite a bit in the beginning because your body is used to getting energy sources all the time. Thanks to the easy availability of food, most of us often eat even when we are not hungry.

Binge eating is a serious problem. Your body may resist fasting and will force you to eat, however, do not worry, this will last only in the beginning, and you will soon be able to tackle it. Whether you do the 16/8 fast or the 5:2 fast, your body will resist in the beginning, especially if you are not used to going hungry. Do not think that your body cannot handle this; it is made to handle long periods of hunger. Just stick to the course, and your body will get accustomed to fasting in a couple of days. If you still think that fasting is difficult and is not meant for you, then you can use various things that will help you transition. The best method to prolong your fast is by using caffeine. Caffeine is a well-known appetite suppressor. It can suppress your hunger bangs for long and will leave you feeling fresh and active. It will also keep the pain away, especially when they are at their strongest. Never overdo caffeine, though. Another way to keep from thinking of hunger is by concentrating on other activities. For instance, if you focus on your work instead of focusing on hunger, you will be able to bear with it for a long time. Do fasting and muscles go hand in hand? Many people believe that fasting is bad for their bodies and that they will lose a lot of muscle mass by fasting. This is a misconception, as fasting does not lead to muscle loss directly. When we fast, our body starts breaking glycogen and converts it into glucose for energy. After the body uses up all the glucose, it starts breaking into fats for energy. It is true that extra amino acids, i.e., proteins, can be used by the body for energy as well. The body will rarely use muscles to fuel itself unless you go into starvation mode. People have been fasting for thousands of years. Unless you go without food for weeks or months, you will be safe and will not lose any muscle mass at all. Is there any specific method of breaking fast? There is no specific method of breaking fast, but many people may find it quite difficult. It is a test of how long you can survive without food. When you break the fast, it is necessary to avoid overloading your body. If you overload your body, you may put a lot of pressure on your digestive system, which may lead to various problems, as well. Secondly, many people tend to overeat after breaking the fast. Overeating can put unnatural stress on your body and thus should be avoided as well. Overeating will also counter everything that you have done by fasting and thus making the net total zero. Planning your meals ahead is the best way to avoid these two phenomena. Instead of breaking your fast with high-calorie foods, go for a simple but hearty omelet. Once you have broken your fast, you can later consume your proper (but healthy) meal. Tips for

Intermittent Fasting People find starting fast quite challenging. You can make the whole process a bit simpler by following these tips.

- Drink water regularly.

- Focus on other activities, such as work.

- Drink black tea or black coffee to avoid hunger pangs.

- Find a fasting group online or offline to keep you motivated.

- Instead of giving in to hunger pangs, avoid them.

- Instead of eating a regular diet, go for low-carb options. They will help you tackle hunger. These options are also good for weight loss.

- While some people may see instant results, do not expect them. Give it a month, at least, and you will surely see and feel a difference.

- Break the fast gently.

- Never binge and avoid overeating.

What chapter should give you a great idea on who should and who shouldn't follow intermittent fasting, as you know, achieving autophagy is very important, and to do that we highly recommend you follow intermittent fasting alongside with the alkaline diet or the ketogenic diet. Whichever diet works for you will work with intermittent fasting. what we spoke about the alkaline diet we suggested that you do not eat any meat, however, do not let that stop you if you do not like the alkaline diet simply follow the intermittent fasting ketogenic plan. As it will still yield the results that you are looking for.

Chapter 6: What to Eat?

We will give you some eating ideas which you can follow to see amazing results. Keep in mind that this is simply a recommendation on what type of diet you should follow. We will talk about the alkaline diet, and the ketogenic diet as these diets tend to work the best when it comes to autophagy.

Alkaline Diet

Many people say that the Alkaline water can help you regulate your body's pH level, and prevent many diseases, including cancer. What is alkaline water, exactly? And why is it essential when it comes to following the alkaline diet and getting better results overall. The salty water refers to its pH level; as you know, the pH level measure is how acidic or alkaline you are or the food. The scale ranges from 0 to 14, one being very acidic and 13 being very alkaline, as we told you in the previous chapters with the sweet spot at 7.5 pHs.

Put, the Alkaline water has a higher level of pH level, which will help your body to become more alkaline, increasing your alkaline level and will neutralize your acidic level in the body. This is why many people recommend that you drink alkaline water right after you drink or eat something which is highly acidic to counteract the balance issue and to alkalize your body overall. Fresh drinking water is generally around 7, whereas the alkaline water is typically about 8 or 9 ph. However, the pH level isn't the most important thing when it comes to making alkaline water. Alkaline water must contain alkaline minerals, which will allow it to have higher antioxidants. Hence making it more alkaline and change to your body in a better way when it comes to alkalizing your body.

It isn't always necessary that the water should be higher in the alkaline level; you must make sure that your alkaline body is absorbing the minerals and making it more alkaline. Hopefully, that makes sense, make sure that your body is alkaline not because of the chemical level in the food or drinks, but it is alkaline from the inside. Although there have not been any studies showing that the alkaline diet can be right for you when it comes to making your body more alkaline, there have been some people saying that the alkaline water could make you get rid of many diseases even if you are not following the alkaline diet.

As you guys might know the tap water is not the safest when it comes to drinking, which is why many people who aren't following the alkaline diet and start drinking alkaline water tend to notice better health benefits because there aren't any added chemicals to it. Our tap water can be very polluted, which is why many people resort to bottled water or, more accurately, alkaline water these days to see better health benefits.

Had our tap water been less polluted, we would not be drinking alkaline water to see better results. Just for reference, the tap water is around 7 pH or close to 7 pHs, whereas the alkaline water has to be above 7 pHs to be called the alkaline water. Our bodies do a fantastic job of maintaining blood pH level, which is why it is not recommended by many people to start drinking alkaline water to see better results.

Nonetheless, alkaline water can help you alkalize your body quickly when compared to drinking regular tap water. If your goal is to become alkaline very quickly, alkaline water can help you tremendously as it is already alkalized and therefore will make your body more alkaline throughout the whole day once you start drinking it as we told you previously, if your very acidic, alkaline water can definitely help you become more alkaline. However, if you are not following the alkaline diet, then it will be tough for you to become alkaline overall even if you are drinking alkaline water, so think of the alkaline water more as a supplement to your diet. Sure, the alkaline water will make you more alkaline to a certain degree, but it will not turn you into an alkaline body overall if you are not following the alkaline diet.

Alkaline water is not great just for the alkaline level, and it is even better because of the mineral contents in it. As you know, the tap water does not have as many minerals as we think it does, more specifically, it isn't as clean and is less polluted when compared to alkaline water, which is why most people tend to drink alkaline water, to see better results and to get more gains out of it. But once you do start drinking the alkaline water, make sure that you are drinking it for the right reasons and that you do not have any health conditions, many people who do have kidney conditions or are taking medications to alter the kidney function it can be harmful to them.

Some of the minerals in alkaline water, cannot be healthy for most people if they are taking any medications or are working on some kidney rehab. Which is why it is essential that you ask your doctor before you start drinking alkaline water regularly, you see our body is not accustomed to alkaline water before we start drinking. Unfortunately, we are accustomed to tapping water or the normal water as we get in our country, which is why alkaline water needs to be assessed before you start drinking it for the right reasons. If your healthy male or female, then you should have no problem with alkaline water as you'll see significant benefits out of it; however, if you are taking any medications or under supervision, make sure you consult with your doctor before you start drinking the alkaline water.

Since you have now understood the function of the alkaline water and how it can help you accordingly, let's talk about some of the benefits that you might see from drinking alkalized water. One of the benefits that you will see from drinking alkaline water is the reduced risk of chronic diseases, more specifically, chronic acidosis. If you have a low-grade chronic acidosis then it might help you that you start drinking some of the alkalized water, the study has not been concreting yet, but there is some suggestion showing that it will help you. Another thing the alkaline water helps you with is to help you with improving your overall health.

As we know by now, alkalizing your body will help you with better bodily functions, better digestion, etc. This is why many people recommend they start drinking alkaline water to better yourself. However, you have to remember that if you want to see better results, then you need to make sure that you are following the alkaline diet alongside the consumption of your alkalized water. In fact, many people who are facing certain conditions should avoid excessive mineral intake; as mentioned to you previously, if you have any kidney conditions, then you need to make sure they consult with your doctor before you start drinking any alkaline water. Another thing that the alkaline water can help you with is to improve athletic performance, again this study has not been concrete yet, but many athletes are suggesting that alkalize water has helped them perform for a more extended period at their peak performance. If you are an athlete, then try out the alkaline water and see how it does for you.

Many people suggest that it will help you. However, many athletes say that it does not help them overall, whereas some do say so; it is a gray matter and therefore needs to be found out by the person itself. Finally, there have been many studies showings that alkaline water can help you with digestion health. This is a great study, but it is up in the air when it comes to the alkalized water helping you with digestion. As we told you previously, when you are alkaline, your body will digest food a lot better, which is why many people start on the alkaline diet. So, it just makes sense if you are drinking alkalized water, that you will see better digestion health overall. Now that you are aware of the alkaline water and how to use it properly, let's talk about how to acquire alkaline water for the best results possible. The alkaline water can be very expensive once you start drinking it regularly, which is why we highly recommend that you make your own alkaline water.

If you have more funds to support your alkaline water needs, then, by all means, you can get your own alkalized water. We recommend Essentia, which is 9.5 on the pH level, this is the bottled water you get, which is alkalized and all ready for you. Make sure that you use this water if you are looking to get more alkalized water in your body, however, if your goal is to make your own alkaline water and there are some ways to go about it. The way most people do it is that use normal tap water, they boil it making sure that they get rid of any pollution in the water. Let the water cool down, and then they will add minerals which they can easily be found online that will make the water even more alkaline.

Once they have done that, you will separately put it in a bottle and finally serve it when chilled. Utilizing this method will ensure they get rid of any pollutions in the water, and you will get a better pH level in the water as well. Your pH level should be around 9.2 to 9.5 if you use this method properly, giving you great alkalize water. However, if you live outside North American and European countries. Then there's a high chance that the water that you are getting from the tap is not drinkable, which is why you might have to spend a little bit more money on the alkaline water. Or you can buy machines which are known as water ionizer, which will create alkaline water, and this method is called ionization. This could be an excellent idea for people who are living outside of North America and European countries to get the cheapest water source of the alkaline water.

With that being said, this should help you really understand how the alkaline water truly works and how you can use it for your own benefit. Let's talk about alkaline fruits and how they can help you when it comes to bettering your health. As you know, there are many alkaline fruits, as you can refer to the chapter in the book where the talk about the whole section of which fruits are alkaline and which aren't. You will get a better idea on which fruits will help your body get alkaline even further; just like the water, the alkaline fruits can genuinely help you with all the same benefits which the alkaline water can. In fact, once you combine the alkaline water alongside the alkaline fruits, you will see even better benefits when it comes to getting your body more alkaline and to see better health benefits overall. One of the great things about the alkaline fruits is that it always helps you with the bone density. It is essential that you take care of your bone density as it can cause a lot of issues if you do not, truth be told since you will not be eating a lot of dairies when following the alkaline diet. Getting a certain amount of calcium from your diet will drop down substantially.

Which is why it is highly recommended that you take bone support. You can take supplements, or it can come from the alkaline fruits that you are going to be eating. Many of the alkaline fruits include blueberries, watermelons, kiwi, etc. These fruits are known to help with bone density, which is why it is imperative that you eat these fruits when you are on the alkaline diet to see a better health benefit overall. Remember, the alkaline diet only works in a certain way; you need to have all aspects of this diet in check for it to work. You have to make sure that your diet is perfect, you have to make sure that you are on the alkaline side in the beginning by using the alkaline strips and finally you need to make sure that you are eating fruit to ensure that you are getting alkalized very quickly. With that being said, the take-home message from this chapter is that it does not matter if you drink alkaline water or you eat the alkaline fruit, everything needs to be in proper conjunction when it comes to seeing better results overall.

You need to make sure that you are eating the right food 24/7, this will ensure that you are alkaline throughout the whole day for you to really see the benefits of having an alkaline body overall. Use this chapter as a tool; these tools will only accompany you with the alkaline diet. Do not think that these tools as the end-all to having an alkaline body if you are not following the alkaline diet, everything needs to be proper if you want to make sure these things help you overall. Hopefully, you have understood the magnitude of these tools and how they can help you.

The Ketogenic Diet Breakdown

Remember how in the early chapters we told you one diet which will go well with intermittent fasting, now we're going to talk about it. The ketogenic diet is one of the best foods you can follow when intermittent fasting, and there's a reason why. When you follow the ketogenic diet, you are using fat for fuel instead of carbohydrates for fuel.

What this will allow you to do is burn more calories throughout the day, the same thing with intermittent fasting. When you are intermittent fasting, you are burning fat for fuel instead of glycogen for fuel, which is why most people suggest ketogenic diet when following intermittent fasting. Now there are a couple of things to consider when following intermittent fasting and ketogenic diet together. In the beginning, it will feel tough for you to follow a ketogenic diet and intermittent fasting along, which is why we recognize slowly add ketogenic diet to your fasting protocol once you get used to intermittent fasting.

The way ketogenic diet works is straightforward when you are following the ketogenic diet, you are not eating any carbs, and you are only eating high-fat moderate protein. When you eat high-fat moderate protein, eventually, your body goes into something called the ketosis. How to get into the ketosis your body with only use energy from fats instead of glycogen Which is why it goes well with intermittent fasting. It will help you burn more calories throughout the day, more specifically, burn more fat throughout the day when you follow the ketogenic diet together. When you follow the ketogenic diet, you make your body produce more ketones, what ketones do is allow your body to use fat for energy instead of anything else. In the next section, we will talk more about ketones and how they work.

More About Ketones

For people that do not know what ketones are, ketones are water-soluble molecules that are produced by the liver and fatty acids. When you are not eating enough food, which includes carbohydrates, your body will go into starvation mode, and once it goes into the starvation mode, it will start using your ketones for energy.

When you have higher levels of ketones in your body will start using any stores available in your body to convert it into energy, there are many ways to check if you are producing enough ketones. There's one year until she can get from any drug store, and it will show you if you are producing enough ketones or not. Just remember that for you to be in the ketogenic diet, you need to be producing enough ketones and be in ketosis.

Moreover, once you are in ketosis, you will start using fat for energy instead of glycogen for energy. When you mix that up with intermittent fasting, you have a recipe for success to lose body fat. Here's the thing when you are falling intermittent fasting you are increasing your ketones in your body. Moreover, when you add a ketogenic diet to the equation, you are further enhancing your chances are boosting ketones in your body. There's nothing else to know about ketones, other than to find out what they do to your body.

Intermittent Fasting and Ketogenic Diet

As you know, when you follow intermittent fasting, you are burning a lot more calories, and therefore it will allow you to burn fat. When you combine a ketogenic diet with intermittent fasting, you will be burning more fat since you do not have to burn any glycogen stores in your bloodstream.

This is why intermittent fasting is one of the best ways to go about burning fat, and once you add a ketogenic diet into conjunction, there is no stopping. There are a couple of things to consider when you are picking out the right method of ketogenic diet protocols, one of the things you need to make sure is the ability to eat food during your eating window. You have to remember that you are still following intermittent fasting, meaning you can't mess that up.

As we have said before, you need to ease into the diet and make sure that you are losing weight at a reasonable rate without noticing any other side effects related to intermittent fasting and keto. One thing you might see when following a ketogenic diet is something called keto flu. This might happen because you are ready for it, so make sure that if you do notice symptoms such as vomiting or lack of strength in the gym. Then you need to consult with your doctor, as we said previously, consult with your doctor before you start any diet or nutrition plan.

Chapter 7: Things to Avoid

The right diet, exercise, fasting, and rest are something you will know when you lock onto your need for autophagy. This need could alter over time, or it may be that you do not need every aspect of it in the same way for the rest of your life. All of the research on autophagy has shown that you do not need to do it every day, but you may find times in the course of your life that you will need or want to activate it on a daily basis. You may lose all the weight you set for your goal, using all four components, but will need to adjust your approach to autophagy once that goal is reached. Life is long and changes daily. There will never be any diet, form of exercise, or fasting ritual that has to stay the same forever unless you are practicing these experiences for religious purposes. We grow, we transform, we change, for our whole lives and so should the food we eat, the kind of exercise we get, how often we fast, and what kind of rest is best under the circumstances.

We do not have the perfect relationship with these factors in a perfect way on all days of the year; we will ebb and flow and need to understand our responsibility to ourselves to pay attention, especially if you want to use autophagy regularly to enhance your health and renewal. Significant research on the overall impact of prolonged autophagy has not been known yet; however, many improvements are being seen and experienced in the overall health of those who include performance autophagy activation in their regular health plans. You can guide yourself along the way using the ideas laid out in these chapters to help you determine the focus of your needs for inducing autophagy.

Let your cells do the dirty work while you plan the routine, and handle the steps and instructions for initiating an autophagic response. Allow for some room to grow and shift. You do not have to follow these guidelines to a T; you can experiment and explore different ways of doing it that work best for your personal, optimal health. Renewal is easy when you bring the right ingredients to the table. This chapter will give you the steps you need to change your diet, exercise, fasting routine, and resting time in order to fully enhance autophagy.

The four categories together promote the ideal healing platform. Remember, the recipe is in your hands, and you have the power to heal.

Right Diet

Taking what you know about how autophagy works and how to activate it, you can begin with the first important steps to creating that internal response. The next steps will give you the approach you need to shift and transition into the right diet. The right diet will initially be a keto-diet for the best autophagic response and weight loss, depending on your goals. A modified diet down the road will be beneficial as well; keeping your body healthy means listening and responding to its needs. A long-term keto diet can be adjusted to allow for more carbohydrates. To begin a ketosis meal plan, you need to ease into it, as you would ease into a period of fasting. The reason for this is that when you immediately stop eating all the foods you are used to eating, such as bread, pasta, sugar, fruit, and many other items, you can enter a shock phase. For some, it can feel like illness, and there can be headaches, cravings, and fatigue. It can feel a lot like the flu. Your body has been eating certain foods for a while, and to suddenly deprive the body of these things can create an inflammatory response. To create a smoother transition from your current eating habits to a keto diet, you will need to break it down into phases and allow for some time.

Week 1 will be the first phase of transition, eliminating some of the foods that you need to avoid to create ketosis.

Week 2 will be the second phase of further elimination and increase in fat and protein. Here is a breakdown of what that may look like:

Elimination of alcohol, unhealthy fats like canola oil, vegetable oil, mayo, margarine, imitation butter, all processed, low-fat foods, condiments that contain sugars and carbs Most grains, including pasta, cereal, bread. You can keep small quantities of grains, like rice, quinoa, and barley. During this elimination, you are taking away some significant carbohydrates but are still allowed to eat some carbs and sugars found in fruit, starchy vegetables, legumes, and other sugary foods and beverages, which will prevent a significant body shock.

It could look like this: Monday Breakfast: eggs and bacon with tomato and mushrooms Lunch: Salad with salmon and fruit on the side Dinner: Chicken soup with rice Tuesday Breakfast: yogurt and berries with a tsp of honey and 3tbsp of almond slivers Lunch: BLT on whole-grain bread Dinner: Steak and potatoes with broccoli

Wednesday Breakfast: Fruit bowl with yogurt Lunch: Salad with chicken and quinoa Dinner: 3 bean soup with sausage and veggies Thursday Breakfast: Goat cheese and basil omelet with tomatoes Lunch: Salmon and asparagus cooked in butter and lemon Dinner: Roast chicken with carrots and potatoes Friday Breakfast: Poached eggs with tomatoes and kale Lunch: Codfish with steamed vegetables and butter Dinner: Beef Stew Saturday Breakfast: Fruit and nuts Lunch: Turkey lettuce wraps Dinner: Roasted pork shoulder with vegetables Sunday Breakfast: Eggs and bacon with a spinach feta salad Lunch: Salad niçoise Dinner: Baked Salmon and broccoli This weekly diet starts to prepare you for an even bigger elimination of carbs and sugars, increasing fat and protein. Cooking with healthy fats like olive oil, coconut oil, and avocado oil is encouraged in Phase 1 and should be adhered to in Phase 2. You can also cook with a small amount of butter or clarified butter known as ghee. There are many keto-diet cookbooks that contain specific cooking recipes to help you avoid incorporating any foods that you are working to eliminate. Avoidance of alcohol during phase one is important. Your body converts alcohol into sugar, so it is like drinking glasses or pints of candy. Increase water consumption and try more herbal teas. One of the reported side effects of ketosis is bad breath.

This is caused by ketones being released in the body from burning fat and can be evident in your breath. Rather than chewing sugary gum or sucking on sweet mints or lozenges, try a few cups of peppermint tea between meals. Adding freshly squeezed lemon juice to your glasses of water is a wonderful digestive aid and can help with balancing internal pH levels. You can also use apple cider vinegar in place of lemon juice to create the same effect. Stay away from processed, packaged foods, and try to prepare meals with fresh ingredients for the best results. Let go of all the protein and power bars, all the cookies and snacks, all the pastries, and flavored lattes. Let go of all the bread and baked goods, all the food made with canola oil and corn syrup. This is what you begin to do and give this phase some time. It does not have to be only one week. It may feel more comfortable for you to extend this phase into 2 weeks or more while your body adjusts, and be sure to drink plenty of water throughout.

Eliminate all grains, including any remaining bread, rice, quinoa, etc. All fruit, except small portions of berries. All sugars and sugar additives, including honey and any beverage containing sugar. Legumes—beans, chickpeas, etc. Starchy vegetables like beets, carrots, potatoes, yams, and parsnips. During this elimination, you are further letting go of any remaining carbs and sugars. The standard ketosis diet allows for 5% daily intake of carbs in ratio to your fat and protein consumption. You can get these carbs from berries and some quantities of vegetables. You will be incorporating more of the high fat/high protein foods your body needs to stave off hunger and cravings, allowing your body to enter enhanced stages of weight loss and ketosis. A typical weekly diet with full elimination could look like this: Monday Breakfast: spinach and goat cheese omelet with three eggs Lunch: tuna salad with feta, olive oil, and lots of leafy lettuce greens Dinner: pork chops with kale salad and broccoli Tuesday Breakfast: yogurt and berries Lunch: big green salad with one avocado, cucumber, celery, green bell pepper, cabbage, toasted walnuts, and an olive oil lemon dressing Dinner: salmon and asparagus with butter and lemon Wednesday Breakfast: bacon and eggs with tomato and basil, side salad Lunch: guacamole with celery and cucumber sticks, a handful of nuts Dinner: pesto chicken and roasted broccoli and Brussels sprouts Thursday Breakfast: mushroom, spinach, tomato-basil omelet Lunch: chicken salad lettuce wraps Dinner: steak and eggs with salad Friday Breakfast: poached eggs on an arugula salad with feta and olive oil Lunch: roasted pork loin and steamed veggies Dinner: tilapia cooked in butter with sautéed broccoli, kale, and spinach Saturday Breakfast: yogurt and berries Lunch: toasted nuts, one avocado, smoked salmon and celery sticks Dinner: roasted turkey breast with a side salad Sunday Breakfast: omelet with scallions, mushrooms, cheddar Lunch: salad niçoise Dinner: roast chicken and Brussels sprouts Keep in mind that while cooking for a ketosis diet, if you need snacks between meals, eat nuts and seeds, or another kind of protein snack.

Use healthy oils and clean ingredients. Do not use canned vegetables. Diet has removed sugars, most carbs, and increased proteins and healthy fats. Use ketosis recipes and cookbooks to help you adjust measurements based on your own weight and BMI. Additionally, if you are going to enjoy breakfast or snack items like yogurt and berries, be sure that you are choosing full-fat yogurt that does not contain any added sugars or flavorings. Finding the right supplements for you can also improve the quality of your daily nutrient intake. Many herbal teas are packed with minerals, vitamins, and nutrients. Having a hot cup of tea between meals can stave off hunger, while soothing and warming the belly, helping it to feel full while packing in minerals and antioxidants. Bone broth can be an excellent supplement to some meals as it is very filling and nutrient-dense. Broths can also be useful in phasing out food to begin transitioning into a fasting period. Bone broths are simple and easy to make at home. You can purchase some quality bone broths from the store, but if you are cooking chicken for your ketosis diet, you can freeze the bones until you are ready to make broth and then put them in a crockpot overnight with purified water.

Add some onion and celery for flavor. There are several recipes available for broths, and you can use a variety of bones, not just chicken. Broths are soothing to the intestinal lining, providing a healthy space for nutrient absorption. Adding bone broths into your daily meals can be a huge improvement to your quality of digestion. You can have a cup of broth instead of tea or skip breakfast or dinner and just enjoy a cup of hot broth. Finding ways to enjoy the program your body is undertaking can feel like a challenge at first, but initiating the process is part of the pleasure of starting your journey to healing. A cup of broth or a handful of your favorite nuts can go a long way. Every person is different, weighs a different amount, and has a different health history. Finding the right recipes for you will help you feel like you can satisfy and satiate your hunger. Ketosis diets are in full, popular swing, and there are numerous delicious recipes to keep you on the right track. Engaging in a ketosis diet while enjoying some of the other autophagic activation methods will ensure a whole healing, whole-body process.

Not all the answers to health and wellness or weight loss and muscle health come from just diet and exercise. The connection that autophagy has to overall wellness and optimal body function has been proven through research and studies over the past several years. A great number of autophagic performance results come from the practice of periodic fasting. What can benefit you most during fasting is the planning and organizing of how and when you will fast for autophagic activation.

There are several approaches to fasting, and all of them can be useful at different times for different purposes. The ones that will be most effective for autophagy in combination with the right diet, exercise, and rest will allow for periods of time with no food at all and water consumption throughout. These periods can last as little as 16 hours or as long as three days. A common fasting practice is the 16:8 ratio. What this means is that you eat nothing for 16 hours and eat 2-3 meals within 8 hours. That could look something like this: 7 am—wake up and drink water and tea 12 pm—eat 3 pm—eat 7-8 pm eat 8 pm-12 pm the next day FAST This is what daily fasting looks like, and depending on your hunger levels, you may only need two meals and a snack or just 1-2 meals.

That is something you have to gauge on the day of the fast. This works well because your body is naturally in a fasting state when you sleep. When you wake up, instead of having breakfast right away, you wait until lunchtime to have your first meal and then have until 8 pm to satisfy your hunger. After 8 pm, you can drink water and herbal tea but will avoid food or snack, as well as alcohol. You can repeat this daily for continued benefit. Another method of fasting that permits longer autophagic response is a longer fast, supported by healthy eating and transition on either side of the fast. An example of this type of fast can look like this: Monday: skip breakfast, eat lunch and dinner Tuesday: skip breakfast and lunch, eat dinner Wednesday: very light dinner only Thursday: water fast Friday: water fast Saturday: drink hot tea in the morning, broth midday, a small amount of yogurt Sunday: broth in the morning, light lunch, light dinner Monday: breakfast, lunch, and dinner.

You can extend the length of the water fast to cover more days, or you can water fast for only one day out of the week, depending on your goals and intentions. You may find as you become familiar with the fasting experience that it is easy to shift back to food, without too much discomfort. Another type of fast involves regular eating five days a week, followed by 2 days of very light eating. You may not experience the most optimal autophagic response, but it will be activated by the extreme calorie reduction over the course of the 2 days. When you decide how you want to fast, the right experience for you will be one that can occur at times where you can rest and not work, especially if you are water fasting. Incorporating the right diet and right exercise over the course of a week can look something like this: Monday Breakfast: skip breakfast, Pilates with weights Lunch: tuna salad with feta, olive oil and lots of leafy lettuce greens Dinner: pork chops with kale salad and broccoli Tuesday Breakfast: skip breakfast, yoga Lunch: skip lunch, water with lemon, and a cup of broth Dinner: salmon and asparagus with butter and lemon Wednesday Breakfast: skip breakfast, water with lemon, one-hour stretching Lunch: skip lunch, herbal tea

Dinner: salad (drink water throughout the day) Thursday Water Fast: water throughout the day, resting, meditation Friday Breakfast: skip breakfast, hot tea and yin yoga Lunch: hot broth, small salad with light dressing Dinner: steamed vegetables with butter Saturday Breakfast: omelet with tomato and basil, cardio workout Lunch: toasted nuts, one avocado, smoked salmon, and celery sticks Dinner: roasted turkey breast with a side salad Sunday Breakfast: omelet with scallions, mushrooms, cheddar Lunch: salad niçoise, Calisthenics Dinner: roast chicken and Brussels sprouts

You can repeat this fasting schedule every week and just play around with the recipes and exercise you do, or you can alternate weeks that you are fasting and do a 2-3 day fast twice a month. The right fast for you is something to explore. Working to create optimal autophagy means allowing for periods of zero-calorie intake, not just when you are asleep, so you can enjoy the maximum benefit of deep cellular healing. Find the fast that is right for your body. You may need to do some experimenting to make sure you can incorporate intermittent fasting into your lifestyle, diet, exercise, and rest.

Right Resting Part of healing is allowing periods of time for your body to regenerate. Autophagy is a powerful, internal intelligence. Your body has the power to heal itself, but if you are not offering it the proper time to rest, you will be digging a deeper hole to clean up later. Starting off on the right foot and creating good, healthy habits for wellness is essential to locking down the results you are looking for.

In our current culture, everything is fast-paced, instantly gratified, and we are all plugged in all day long to our devices. Many people have 40-60 work weeks that make it challenging to find time for rest, let alone diet, exercise, and healthy fasting. Bringing your health into focus includes allowing for proper periods of rest. During your experience in activating autophagy, it will be important to organize the time for your body to rest. Rest is important after significant exercise. When you strain and stress your body, it requires time to recover and repair microscopic damage to the muscle fibers and tissues.

When you eat a meal that is filling, it is helpful to enjoy a period of rest after to allow your body the proper amount of time to digest. Your body can focus on digestion better if you offer it the rest to do so. Fasting is something that can temporarily lower your energy since you are not ingesting any calories. It is common to experience some fatigue under these circumstances. It is a great opportunity to incorporate rest for your body while it is fasting. Imagine, too, on the microscopic level, when you are resting, your body is undergoing great healing, transformation, and change, performing autophagic response from the intermittent fasting. Many people consume large amounts of sugar and caffeine daily to bump them out of slumps that occur throughout the day, after meals, after long periods of work, or because of lack of sleep the night before. If you replace your caffeine and sugar doses with moments or periods of rest throughout the day, you will aid your body in a much healthier way, eliminating the need for caffeine and sugar altogether.

Sugar is the antithesis of a healthy diet and optimal autophagic performance and should be avoided anyway if you are planning on activating autophagy. Caffeine is regularly consumed by most people, and it is not discouraged in the majority of diets. The longer-term effects of daily caffeine intake can be as detrimental to your body as any other stimulant or toxin. Successful autophagic performance does not need caffeine and like other foods and beverages that hinder health. It should be avoided and replaced with herbal teas, water, and other non-caffeinated beverages. You can ultimately rest better without it, and if you are getting the rest you need, you will not need caffeine at all.

The right rest comes with experimentation, awareness of your needs, listening to your body, and responding to it when it is asking for rest. Incorporating the right rest will fluctuate depending on day to day life, activities, exercise, diet, schedule, and more. Rest is vital to supporting optimal autophagic performance. All four components together bring about a level of health that will deliver clear results that you can see and feel. Activating autophagy through the combination of the right diet, exercise, fasting, and rest is the key to a long and healthy life.

Chapter 8: How to Make
This a Lifestyle

In this chapter, we will talk about how to make autophagy lifestyle so that it is very easy for you to follow in the long-term. Believe it, or not many people have issues following has died, the reason why they have issues following the status because it can be very hard and confusing. After reading this book, you should have a clear idea of many ways to follow intermittent fasting, alkaline diet, or ketogenic diet to achieve your goals of autophagy. However, understanding the core benefits when it comes to keeping a long-term is another thing. If you can keep following a certain plan for the long-term, not only will they see better results when it comes to Better Health and overall well-being, but it will be easy for you to make this a lifestyle. In this chapter, we will give you certain ways for you to start building up habits so that you can actually start making this plan a habit.

Many of you are facing the issue of self-discipline, and quite frankly, it isn't your fault. Self-discipline is something that has been not paid attention to for a long time now, and many think that self-discipline takes a lot of dedication and encouragement to get it up and to run. However, the truth is that it is very easy, and anyone can achieve proper self-discipline. In this chapter, we're going to talk about how to build self-discipline, overall helping you to become better at whatever it is that you are trying to achieve. However, before we get into how you can achieve optimal self-discipline, let's talk about what self-discipline people are currently doing. Self-disciplined people do not tend to spend much time enjoying things that they know are detrimental to their health. they have a very positive outlook on life, which allows them to stay focused and stay positive on the things which they're trying to achieve. remember that, I will give you all the tips necessary to become more self-disciplined, but you have to get into the mindset of successful people to achieve optimal self-discipline.

The first thing when it comes to achieving optimal self-discipline would be to know your weaknesses. we all have weaknesses, whether it's socializing on Facebook or eating foods that we shouldn't be eating. We are all addicted to something which does not support our goals and health, and You need to acknowledge your self-destroying habits. Really understand what gets you to do bad things, which cause you to become less disciplined and more procrastinating; once you acknowledge all your shortcomings and things that cause you to become less self-discipline, then you can start to really born on those certain habits and fix them.

The first thing you need to do is figuring out all your shortcomings, and then you can move on to the next steps. Once you manage to figure out all your self-discipline issues, the next thing you need to do is make sure that you remove all the Temptations around you. The best way to describe it is out of sight and out of mind if you are around certain things that make you do things would cause you to become more self-discipline then you need to get rid of them. For instance, if you like unhealthy snacks and you are trying to lose weight, then you need to get rid of those snacks as soon as possible. Essentially, it would be best if you got rid of all the things which are holding you back in order to achieve optimal success and self-discipline. The next thing when it comes to achieving self-discipline Optimal Health, would be the set clear goals and have an execution plan. If you have hopes of achieving self-discipline and overall success, then you need to have an execution plan with detailed results and goals. You cannot accomplish things you need to have a set plan and set goals that will allow you to get there.

Overall, if you do not have goals or set plans to achieve your goals, then you will derail and cause you to become a lot less self-discipline overall. A clear plan would be something that shows you each step on how you are going to achieve something, for example, let's just say you want to lose a certain amount of weight then chances are you need to have a certain guy plant in a certain workout regimen which will allow you to get there.

Every successful person uses this technique to achieve optimal success in their field, so make sure they have a clear idea of what you are trying to achieve and how you are going to get there come up with a detailed plan. However, you have to realize that no one's born with optimal self-discipline; we build it. Think of self-discipline as a skill, and you have to build up the skill by practicing it every day, which will help you achieve optimal success and overall well-being.

We understand that doing certain tasks require a lot of self-discipline, so slowly build up to a certain amount of work every day, which will help you to become a lot more self this one of the things you are trying to achieve. For example, let's say you are into working out in trying to lose a certain amount of weight, start with three times a week of working out 30 minutes a day and then slowly increase your workouts as you go become a lot more difficult to achieve. This Progressive overload up optimal success and self-discipline will allow you to become a lot more self-discipline and every other aspect of your life. think of self-discipline as working out.

If you want to achieve better self-discipline, then do your daily diligent of doing tasks that are important to you in order to build better self-discipline. Speaking of doing small things that will help you become more self-disciplined, you need to create new habits every day and keep them simple if you want to achieve overall self-discipline. in previous chapters, we have talked about how to achieve new habits if you want to be more self-disciplined, then you need to start achieving your habits in order to get to your goals.

You have to remember the fact that it takes a lot of work ethic to get where you want to get to, which means you need to start building your habits, and you need to keep them simple. We can understand that building new habits can be daunting at first, but if you take many steps and eventually get to the point where you are, then habits will seem a lot easier to build. This tip is one of the most important tips you will hear in this book, and you want to achieve optimal success, then you need to start building habits right now.

Another thing would be when it comes to achieving optimal discipline; it would be to become a lot healthier. Studies show that healthy people have a lot more self-discipline with the work that they're trying to do. If your goal is to be more self-disciplined in to achieve a lot more goals, then you need to start eating healthier and start feeling healthier. you might have heard the phrase health is wealth, it is true you need to be a lot healthier for optimal functioning, optimal functioning will equal to better self-discipline. You need to start working out if you are right now, and you need to start eating a lot healthier and more frequently in order to stay filled for the day.

Make sure whatever it is that you are doing is healthy and always ask a doctor or get a piece of medical advice before you start anything. Another way to ensure that you get optimal willpower, it's not to limit yourself. There have been studies showing that people who limit their selves or talked themselves into believing that they do not have enough willpower, will not have enough willpower in the long run.

If you have any beliefs in your mind that you are not strong enough to do something or you do not have the willpower to do something, then chances are you will not achieve that goal, and you will be held back. Get rid of all the disbelief that you have in your mind before you start anything, whatever you set your mind to it you can achieve so make sure that if you believe that you do not have enough willpower to keep something then get rid of it and start working on the project right now.

This will allow you to become a lot more successful at your work, and overall, get stronger will power. Also, having a back-up plan is crucial. Many psychologists believe that if you give yourself a back-up plan, you will be a lot more discipline and have a higher will power, for example, let's say you are doing some work and you feel like you can't get it done today then make sure you much time tomorrow to get it done. Do not force yourself into doing something that you know you can't complete; developing will power is like working out; you need to build it up slowly in order to see optimal results and success. Many will disagree with this, but I will tell you this is having a back-up plan, in the beginning, will help you to be a lot more focused, so you work and actually get a lot of your work done hence increasing your willpower in the long run.

It would be best if you rewarded yourself whenever you achieve some success. Rewarding yourself has shown to increase willpower in the long run, we need to have an incentive if you want to increase your willpower. if you have no incentive to achieve something, then chances are you will not get there, hence yourself some short-term goals and once you achieve them to reward yourself. A classic example of this method would be something called a cheat day. Many people were falling a diet or working out, tend to have a cheat day once they've achieved one whole week of clean eating. This can be used in any platform, so make sure that you are worthy soft every time you achieve a certain milestone to keep yourself going and to get more willpower in you. Also remember, to forgive yourself if you have any mishaps.

We are humans, and the chances of us giving up or two mess up on certain things are very high, especially in the beginning. Do not beat yourself to it; if you make a mistake, that's fine, then keep going on, and you will achieve the goals you are trying to achieve. Remember, every successful person has failed in the short term, do not worry about some mishaps here and there. If you made a mistake, that's fine; simply forgive yourself and move on and make sure whatever mistake you have made has been forgiven and recognized by you. This will help you to move forward and not to make any mistakes. This brings us to the end of the chapter, make sure that you follow all the tips and tricks on this book, especially in this chapter.

If you want to achieve more self-discipline, think of it as a workout, not only will this help you to increase your willpower slowly, but it will help you increase it at an optimal level. also remember, willpower takes a lot of work and effort every successful person what was not born with optimal will power. If you want to be successful and achieve many things, then make sure that you were going to increase your will power by working hard and to slowly increase it by following the steps listed in this book.

Do not forget to read all. The previous chapters to make this chapter even more useful to you, and this will help you to become a lot more successful in the long run to make sure that you read all the previous chapters that we've talked about when it comes to building habits and all the above. Finally, make sure they believe in yourself; this is the biggest holding back thing that most people are facing when they're trying to achieve optima will power. you can do it, just like everybody did.

How to Deal With Interruptions

Many of you are with many interruptions throughout the day. The chances of you facing interruptions during work or anything that you are doing very important is quite high. This is why in this chapter, we are going to talk about how to deal with interruptions, the proper way as there are many ways to deal with interruptions, we're going to talk about the right way to deal with it. Now they're all so many ways to deal with it the right way, and it depends on the situation how deep you are into an interruption. With that being said, it is important that you do not get interrupted if you want to be successful in life. Whatever you have to do, make sure that you are not interested, but then again, it is a lifestyle that does happen with us, so without further ado, let's talk about how to deal with interruptions the right way. This will be more attracted to people who are getting interrupted by people who are bothering them at work. The first thing you need to do when you are getting interrupted is to just let it go; everybody gets interrupted here and there, so the chances of you getting interrupted are high as well. Make sure if it happens the first time simply Let It Go and then move on to your work. You have to realize that, for you to obtain an optimal workday, you will have to work in a nice little place with no one is going to be there for 8 hours, and for most people, that isn't the case. However, it's a bother you the next time around tell them politely stop interrupting you. This will give you a clear idea of whether they're going to drop you again, and you will send out the message to the people are interrupting you that you are serious about not getting interrupted. The third time be a little bit more aggressive when it comes to telling them not to run up to you, be very find about how you feel about you getting interrupted and tell them that you are trying to achieve something which is quite important to you so you would appreciate it if they didn't interrupt you.

Finally, if they interrupt you the four-time then deliver more aggressive about it and tell them that you are not appreciating how they're bothering you when you are working. this is how to deal with interruptions when you are being interrupted at work by a certain person, just make sure that in the beginning, you were nice about it, and if they continue on, then you need to tell them more abruptly and more aggressively

Now you have to remember that interruptions can come from any time and any place, this is a very crucial thing to understand when you are trying to achieve success with your diet or work in general. Make sure that you follow all these steps above so that you get a clear idea of how to set your day accordingly so that you see success in the field that you are looking for. Remember, these tips are not just about following a certain diet, but these tips will help you in the long term to set up your life the way you want it to be. This chapter was to show you how to be successful in anything in life, not just following intermittent fasting or autophagy.

It is very important to understand these topics as a can help you in life to be successful. Many people do not talk about this topic, especially in a diet book, but the truth is in order to be successful when following a diet, you need to be productive, and you need to have the willpower to do so. This is one of the biggest misconceptions people have, is that reading a book will give you the success you need. Sure, the book will guide you to where you want to be; however, it is your job to do whatever it takes to achieve success and greatness and whatever it is you are trying to achieve. Overall, the main thing to take home from this chapter is that having good willpower and knowing when to stop will give you the success you are looking to achieve. I know this chapter might have been boring to you, but trust me, this chapter perhaps the most important chapter you will ever read when it comes to bettering your chances of success. When following this plan, or any plan in general. Bettering your health is just as important as your work life, and it is very important to treat it as such. It is a part of your life, which revealed numerous amounts of results if you keep doing great things to take care of it.

Conclusion

Thank you so much for purchasing the book *Intermittent Fasting and Autophagy: A Step by Step Beginners Guide for Weight Loss, Build Muscle, Detox Your Body and Boost Your Energy Through the Process of Metabolic Autophagy for Women and Men*. As you can tell, after reading this book, we went through a lot of things when it comes to autophagy and how to follow the right way to see the proper results.

Keep in mind that when it comes to this method, you have to make sure that your diet is perfect or at least good to see results. As you read this book, we talked about intermittent fasting and how it can help you to see your results from autophagy. Also, a ketogenic diet can help you tremendously with autophagy.

You are keeping that in mind, it is now in your hands to decide what kind of diet you are going to be following and how you are going to get there based on the knowledge provided to you in this book. What we did a great job in this book was to help it be more customized. More specifically, how to figure out how to pick out the right plan for your needs and how to achieve the true autophagy that you have been looking for. With that being said, we conclude this chapter. Thank you so much for reading it till the end, and we hope you enjoyed this book.

www.ingramcontent.com/pod-product-compliance
Lightning Source LLC
Chambersburg PA
CBHW070354220526
45467CB00001B/370